LIFE EXTENSION

A PRACTICAL GUIDE FOR A LONG LIFE

Adding Vitality
Through Life Choices

Don Durrett

(Fourth Edition, November 2019)

Copyright © 2017 by Donald David Durrett
All rights reserved.

ISBN: 978-1-4276-5600-1

www.DONDURRETT.com

BOOKS BY DON DURRETT

The Demise of America

Kern County: The Path to Secession and a New Constitution

How to Invest in Gold and Silver: A Complete Guide with a Focus on Mining Stocks

A Stranger From the Past

Conversations With an Immortal

Finding Your Soul

Finding Your Soul Workbook

New Thinking for the New Age

Spirit Club

Last of the Gnostics

The Gathering

Ascension Training

Team Creator

Longevity is a choice,
unless you are lucky.

– Don Durrett

Contents

Introduction vii

Chapter One
Exercise 1

Chapter Two
Rest 11

Chapter Three
Take Supplements 17

Chapter Four
Reduce Stress 21

Chapter Five
Eat Well 27

Chapter Six
Drink Well 55

Chapter Seven
No Drugs or Chemicals 59

Chapter Eight
Plan to Live to 100 61

Chapter Nine
Extreme Methods 65

Introduction

Today someone emailed me a short list of things to do to live a long life. I emailed him back with my own personal list. I realized that each item on my list could be a chapter in a book. I started thinking about whether I wanted to write it. Why not? It's a subject that I am passionate about and a lifestyle I have followed for over thirty years.

A few years ago, my cousin tried to get me to write a book about how to eat healthily. I turned him down and said that it had already been done by dozens of writers. Now I can satisfy his desire by including it in a more comprehensive book about health. Longevity is really about holistic health and all the areas of our life that impact our health.

I've been taking care of myself since my early twenties. I remember my dad making fun of my healthy diet when I was in college. He thought healthy diets were ridiculous. I joined a gym when I was nineteen and still go on a weekly basis. I never stopped going. I started jogging in my twenties and have run in several half marathons.

So, diet and exercise started early for me, and have been a part of my lifestyle for quite some time. I turn fifty-seven this month, but I look forty-five. Quite often, people are surprised when I tell them my age. I'm five feet ten inches tall and weigh 150 pounds. I've never been overweight. People tell me that I need to eat more and gain weight, but I know that my weight is ideal for a long life, which is my goal.

I am a spiritual writer and spirituality is very important to me. I believe that spirituality and health go hand in hand. In other words, if you have health issues, then your spirituality will be impacted. For this reason, I try to not allow health to block my spiritual growth. You will find that most monks eat a healthy diet. Why? Because the body is a vessel that holds the soul. It should be a sacred temple that is respected.

That's my motivation. It does not need to be yours. Everyone needs their own motivation and determination for attempting to extend their life beyond the average expected lifespan. However, without some type of strong motivation, the results will be less than optimal. Longevity is not something that is easily achieved.

When I say longevity, I'm not talking about simply living beyond the average lifespan. Just making it to old age is not enough. The key is the quality of your health throughout your life. What you want to extend is your vibrancy. You want to equate longevity with vitality. When you turn eighty, you want to feel much younger. In my opinion, that can only be accomplished through effort, or perhaps, genetic luck.

My focus on spirituality led me to strive for longevity in all aspects of my life. I will likely live until I am 100, and I plan to. Not because of genetics, but because of a healthy lifestyle. If you follow a similar lifestyle guided by this book's suggestions, then the odds of extending your life are extremely high. If you want longevity, then read this book and take it to heart.

I believe that anyone can add five to ten years to their life if they begin following the recommendations in this book. Even if you consider yourself old, it's not too late. The key to success will be adhering to the recommendations in all nine chapters. If you skip one, your potential for longevity is diminished.

In many respects, living a long life is the result of our genes. However, it is my belief that longevity is a choice, unless you are lucky. We can hope to have a long life, but only those who are lucky or those who are proactive will have one. Today, most people die long before old age, or perhaps their vibrancy is diminished before old age. Both of my parents died relatively young from illness. I am nearly certain they could have extended their lives by using the suggestions discussed in this book before they got ill. Most illnesses, including cancer, can be prevented with a bit of effort (at least that is my belief). Of course, it's not easy and requires a new lifestyle.

In addition to a new lifestyle, you will need to devote more resources (money) toward your overall health. The cost of quality food and a steady flow of supplements can require a substantial increase to your monthly budget.

The message of this book is two-fold. First, a long and vibrant life is achievable. Second, we know how to do it. The hard part is wanting it. I'm sure that many of you will read one of these chapters and say, "I can't do that." However, if you truly want to add years to your life, and extend the number of vibrant years you will live, then yes, you can.

One final point. I want to define what I mean by a long or an extended life. I consider a long life to be at least ninety years of age. The average lifespan is around seventy-five to eighty years of age. Anyone who lives significantly beyond this age is living an extended life, either by genetics or through lifestyle choices.

Living a long life should not be your goal. Instead, it should be living a long, vibrant life. You want to extend your vibrancy and vitality well beyond what is considered normal. If you can do that, then a long life will be the result. There are people today in their eighties who are as vibrant as those who are decades younger. That should be your goal.

Don Durrett 3/9/2017

Chapter One

EXERCISE

For the majority of people, exercise is not enjoyable, and not something that they do on a regular basis. If you fall into this category, then it is time to change your habits and your attitude regarding exercise. You need to perceive it as something that is necessary. Why? Because exercise might be the most important thing that you can do to extend your life.

The number one indicator for human longevity is our telomeres. These are caps at the end of each of our chromosomes. As we age, our telomeres shorten and our cells stop regenerating. Once they are gone, so are we. There is actually a company that will tell you how old you are in telomere years.

Science has proven a direct link between exercise and the rate that our telomeres shorten. Those who exercise regularly have telomeres that shorten at a slower rate, showing increased telomerase activity. So, we have proof. Exercise will extend your life.

Not only does exercise promote life extension, but it is perhaps the best way to avoid the doctor's office. People will brush their teeth twice a day and floss in order to avoid going to the dentist, but rarely do they exercise to avoid going to the doctor. The best thing you can do for promoting health is exercise. Nothing is better as a preventative medicine.

Did you know that running can potentially add three years to your life? That has been proven with scientific studies. If you run two hours a week, it will add about fourteen hours to your life. If you are a runner, you are adding about one month to your lifespan each year, until you max out at about three additional years. Researchers found that running over two hours a week does not provide any additional lifespan benefit.

If running is extending our lifespan, then surely all forms of exercise are doing the same thing. In fact, I would submit that multiple forms of exercise have a multiplier effect on extending our lives.

The benefits of exercise are extensive. Here is a partial list:
1) Keeps you strong and vibrant.
2) Helps control your weight and blood sugar levels.
3) Good for your brain (memory, focus, concentration) and mental health.
4) Enhances quality of sleeping.
5) Slows aging (increases mitochondrial function and telomerase activity).
6) Prevents illness.
7) Prevents injuries.
8) Good for your skin.
9) Gives you energy.
10) Reduces stress (increases dopamine levels).

Wow, that's an amazing list. You would think nearly everyone would exercise after reading that list. Sadly, only about twenty percent of adults exercise enough to proactively extend their lives. It's time for you to join that group.

The key to success with exercise is making it a part of your lifestyle. It has to be a lifestyle choice, the same as deciding to brush your teeth twice a day. Once the choice has been made, it has to become a part of your routine, without fail. Then, when your doctor asks, "How often do you exercise?" You can say, "On a regular basis."

Chapter One: Exercise

Do you think you can do that? If not, then it's probably time to put this book back on the shelf. Why? Because without exercise, the odds of a long, vibrant life are severely reduced. There is a reason that this is the first chapter. We might as well get the bad news out of the way. If you want to be vibrant well into your eighties, it's not likely to happen without regular exercise.

Okay, now that you have decided to include regular exercise into your lifestyle, how are you going to carry it out? You have several options. Here is a partial list:

1) Jogging or running.
2) Cycling or an elliptical-type machine.
3) Swimming.
4) Walking or hiking (preferably at a brisk pace or incline).
5) Workouts with weights.
6) Isometric/calisthenic workouts (push-ups, pull-ups, etc.).
7) Aerobic workouts.
8) Sports (that raise your heart rate).
9) Yoga.

If you have not tried everything listed, then you are probably not sufficiently motivated to have a healthy body. It's time for you to have an attitude adjustment and begin taking your body more seriously. Because without sufficient motivation, it's impossible to maintain a consistent exercise routine. And what could be a better motivation than wanting a healthy, vibrant, long life? If you think about it, what's more important than your health? Are you motivated now?

One of my favorite movie scenes is from *Man on Fire*, in which Denzel Washington helps Dakota Fanning win a swimming race.

He asks her, "Trained or untrained?" and she replies, "Trained." He is basically asking her if she is motivated to win.

Your job is to find an exercise that you prefer, or several. The key is to be consistent. Ideally, you want to raise your heart rate for an extended period of at least twenty minutes, twice a week. When you raise your heart rate, you are truly exercising. This is the real deal. Doing some form of workout with weights or calisthenics can raise your heart rate, but they usually fail to achieve your aerobic goal. For this reason, I advise that you find some form of aerobic exercise that you like.

I have always lifted weights and jogged. This dual-themed exercise program has worked very well for me. It achieves both my goal of strength and aerobic exercise. What I have learned is that you do not have to do that much for real results. When I was younger, I used to run long distances of six miles or more. I also used to work out in the gym with weights for an hour or longer. I have found out with experience and research that I was wasting my time.

There is very little added benefit once you have raised your heart rate for twenty to thirty minutes, and the same goes with strength workouts. The fact is, less is better. It's much better to increase your intensity and shorten your workouts. Some people have shortened their strength workouts to ten minutes and received enormous benefits. However, I recommend twenty to thirty minutes for both aerobic and strength workouts. You can use this same time frame for swimming, a stationary bike, or an elliptical machine.

Interval workouts have shown, in studies, to be the most beneficial. For example, it's much better to exercise at a high intensity, rest, and then repeat. This is better for your body than swimming, jogging, or cycling at the same even pace throughout your workout. It's a more intense workout, but also much better for you. Repeat after me: intense, rest, intense, rest. That's what interval training is all about.

One optimal method of exercise is raising your heart rate significantly and then using short rest periods, thereby preventing your heart from returning to its normal resting heart rate. Using this method, you can keep your heart rate elevated for an extended period. For example, you can run (or swim or cycle) a lap as fast as you can, and then take a short rest. However, do not rest long enough for your heart to return to its normal rate. Then run (swim or cycle) the next lap at a fast pace. Do this to keep your heart rate elevated for twenty minutes.

Another method I like is to run a mile on a treadmill as fast as I can, then after a very short rest, I do a weight exercise at a high intensity. I do another short rest, and repeat the weight exercise. During my rest breaks, I monitor my heart by feeling it pounding in my chest to ensure that it remains elevated. Before my heart can return to its normal heart rate, I do the next weight exercise. This may sound ultra-intense, but it really isn't. All you are doing is limiting your rest periods and pushing yourself a bit. I have found that it isn't that much more difficult than a normal weight workout with very little heart rate elevation.

So, there you go. You only need to exercise for twenty to thirty minutes twice a week to extend your life. That's all that is required. You can extend workouts to forty minutes, or even an hour if you want. Plus, if you add a third or fourth day that's even better. However, anyone who is exercising five days or more is just having fun. From a health and longevity perspective, it's overkill. In fact, too much exercise can lead to chronic injuries, such as knees and shoulders.

Researchers have found that the maximum health effect for the body is running two hours a week. That probably applies to all methods of exercise to some extent. Once you reach a certain level of exercise for a week, the benefits to the body diminish dramatically. Basically, you are wasting your time, unless you are trying to compete at some sport. Yes, you can get faster or stronger with extended exercise, but not healthier.

Give your body a minimum of two workouts a week. I personally enjoy my workouts, so I usually try to do four. I break this down into two strength workouts and two aerobic workouts. For my strength workouts, I lift weights for thirty to forty minutes. For my aerobic workouts, I usually run two to four miles, or sometimes I will cycle for one hour. I have also swum a lot of laps in a pool and plan to do more of that in the future.

One idea for you is to do both your strength and aerobic workouts on the same day. Then you only need to exercise twice a week. If you do both for twenty minutes, you will be done in less than an hour. If you are not an exercise person, then I would recommend this routine.

Do not think you can do either aerobic workouts or strength workouts and get the same benefits. You need to do both because they each provide different benefits, and both are important. For women who do not like strength workouts, I would suggest yoga as an alternative.

You may think that you can avoid both aerobic workouts and strength workouts, and still extend your life by being "active." Many people like to perform what I call mild forms of exercise that essentially are neither aerobic nor strength exercises. This would include walking, sports such as golf or bowling, hiking, gardening, etc. These types of exercise are beneficial, but not sufficient because they do not raise your heart rate. If you are serious about extending your life, then a combination of aerobic and strength exercises are the most beneficial.

Chapter One: Exercise

The weekly aerobic exercises are important for the listed reasons at the beginning of this chapter. This is why you want to elevate your heart rate every week. There is one other benefit that I did not list. Over time, your resting heart rate will drop. In fact, it will likely drop more than ten percent and perhaps twenty percent! Most people who do not exercise have heart rates around sixty beats per minute. Mine has been below fifty for many years. That means my heart works twenty percent less than the average person. The more aerobic exercise you do, the more it will drop.

If you are over thirty years of age, then I would do a treadmill stress test with your doctor to ensure that you do not have any blockages. I had one done and it was easy. It only takes about fifteen minutes and you can find out if you have any heart disease or blockages.

For those of you who think you can skip the stress test, I had a friend whose husband died of heart attack while jogging before he was thirty-five. If you have been sedentary and have recently not done very much aerobic exercise, then a stress test can give you the green light. These tests not only provide the okay to exercise intensely, but they validate your diet, and give you peace of mind that your arteries are clear.

* * * * *

There are a few things that I have done for the last thirty years that I highly recommend. The first is sit-ups, both forward and reverse. It is my belief that sit-ups are crucial for keeping your back in good working order. I always do sit-ups either before or after my workout. I have occasionally had lower back pain, but once I do some sit-ups, the pain goes away.

The next thing I have done is to stretch. I stretch before I do sit-ups. I believe that stretching prevents injuries. The areas to stretch are your hips, spine, lower back, groin, hamstrings, and calves. If you remain limber, you can stretch all of these areas in about two minutes with relative ease. I personally have never overstretched, but it is possible to create an injury if you stretch too hard.

You probably haven't thought of stretching your feet, but I recommend stretching your feet tendons using a tennis ball. As you age, the tendons in your feet lose their elasticity. A simple exercise with a tennis ball will stretch your tendons. What you do is stand on a tennis ball in your bare feet and roll it back and forth. Here's how to do it. While standing barefoot, put the ball under your left foot. Use your left hand to brace against a table or chair so that you don't fall down. Put as much weight as possible on the ball and roll it from the back of your foot to the front, and then roll it back. Do this twenty or thirty times for each foot when you wake up in the morning. If you do this, you will keep your foot tendons stretched and elastic. Plus, you won't have any foot pain.

If you think this foot exercise is a waste of time, have someone who is over forty years old stand barefooted on a tennis ball. Most people can't because of the intense pain from a lack of elasticity. If you have this pain, it will quickly go away after you begin daily stretching with a tennis ball. What's amazing is that tens of thousands of people have foot pain and don't know about this simple cure.

When you are stretching out your foot tendons, it is an opportune time to do hand exercises. I have spent thousands of hours on a computer keyboard in my lifetime, and occasionally, I get pain in my hands and wrists. I have found that by squeezing an inexpensive hand grip, thereby strengthening my hands and wrists, it prevents pain. While I stretch my left foot, I squeeze a hand grip with my right hand. I squeeze once for each movement of the tennis ball back and forth. Then, when I stand on my right foot, I move the hand grip to my left hand and repeat the exercise.

These simultaneous exercises accomplish two things at once, and both exercises are easy to do. Since I began doing this, the occasional pain in my hands and wrists has been significantly reduced.

If you do a daily morning exercise with a tennis ball and a hand grip, most of you will prevent any future pain issues with your feet, hands, or wrists. And it will take less than two minutes.

Chapter Two

REST

This chapter could have been titled *Sleep* because sleep is where we get most of our rest. However, sleep is only part of the answer. Most people do not consciously think about getting enough rest. You can get enough sleep and still not get enough rest. If you work all the time, then you are probably not getting enough rest.

Work can wear us out. We work for a paycheck, but we also work around the house. Women often work harder than men because they have more hats to wear. My mom was a working mother and she did all of the shopping and cooked all of the meals. She worked twice as hard as my dad. It's still the same for many working women.

Many people work a significant amount of time without sufficient rest. These long hours of working eventually add up and impact our health. In fact, no one is aware that this burden of working long hours is taking years off of their lifespan. If people who are working all hours of the day could find a way to relax and rest, they could add years to their life.

If this is you, then, perhaps, add more exercise to your life. Your exercise routines can give you a chance to relax. Other ways include spending more time socializing or spending time with family and friends. Find some outlets that take you away from work. Too much work is going to wear you out and impact your longevity.

If you don't have an overwhelming work burden, then your only rest nemesis is getting enough sleep. Some people can live on six hours of sleep, some people even less. However, they are the exceptions. Most of us begin to age prematurely from sleep deprivation. Most of us need at least seven hours of sleep, and some of us need eight, or more. This is something that you have to learn on your own. Everyone should know what their ideal sleep requirement is, and then try to consistently hit that number.

One key to longevity and an extended life is knowing your sleep number and then hitting that number. Moreover, to keep your body rested, you do not want to confuse it by living on a variable sleep schedule. If you are consistent, then your body will be consistently rested.

Now, everything I have said about rest is common sense. However, just like exercise, it is a lifestyle choice. You choose to be rested. It's a decision that you personally make. Most people have the philosophy that "I only live once, and I'll sleep when I die." Well, those are not the people who live an extended life.

I do not have good genetics for a long life on my father's side, but on my mother's side, my grandfather lived until he was ninety-one, and died of emphysema. I think he might have made it to 100 if he hadn't been a smoker. At age ninety-one, emphysema was his only health issue. He was a man who always got his rest. He was a farmer and always went to bed early. I honestly believe his rest habits extended his life.

Stick to your sleep schedule and stay rested. Your health will benefit, and your potential for life extension will be enhanced.

The key to rest is to stay rested, and to have a routine that keeps you rested. If you get run down and tired, then take the time to recharge and do not continue in that state. Better yet, do not allow yourself to get run down. Know your limits and adhere to them. Stay rested.

Here are the top five reasons for a reduced lifespan (less than average):

Chapter Two: Rest

1) Cigarettes.
2) Drug and alcohol abuse.
3) Obesity.
4) Illness.
5) Lack of sleep.

The first four items are obvious, but what is a lack of sleep doing on that list? Until recently there had been very little research done regarding sleep. Now we know that the body is actually very active during sleep, especially the brain. The process of rejuvenation during sleep is quite complex. It turns out that the brain does just as much work when we are asleep as when we are awake. Moreover, a deficient amount of sleep can be detrimental to both our health and longevity.

It's amazing that people will eat a healthy diet and then deprive themselves of sleep. Or, consistently exercise and then forget to sleep.

Find out how much sleep you need so that you are not drowsy during the day, and then consistently sleep that many hours. Normally that is at least seven hours, with some people needing a bit less or a bit more. I personally need at least eight, and wish I could get by on less. I can get by on less than eight, but I can tell that I am not completely refreshed during the day. A refreshed body will tell you your optimal number of hours of sleep.

One thing to be aware of about sleep is that not all sleep is equal. There is something called rapid eye movement (REM) sleep, which is different than deep sleep. The body cycles in and out of REM sleep throughout the night, and you only REM sleep twelve to fifteen minutes per hour. The more hours of sleep you get, the more cycles of REM you receive. The average person gets about ninety minutes of REM sleep each night.

Because REM sleep is the most refreshing, you want to eliminate anything that can prevent it. The first thing to eliminate is excessive light and sound. Find out if you are sensitive to light by making your bedroom completely pitch black for two weeks and see if it helps. I did this test and found no difference. I actually prefer to sleep with some light in the room.

You can also try using ear plugs and a sleep mask and see if they help. Next, make sure the room temperature is between 68 and 77 degrees. And do not consume caffeine, chocolate, alcohol, sugar, or heavy foods within four hours of bedtime. Lastly, consider the air quality in the room.

Many of us are highly concerned about the quality of our water and then neglect the quality of the air in our homes. Air quality can impact both our sleep and our health. The first thing to check is the humidity level. You can buy a humidity tester for $10 on Amazon.com. You want your level to be around fifty percent for sleeping. For those of you who live in areas of high humidity, you can control your bedroom humidity by purchasing a dehumidifier. And for those of you in dry climates, you can add a humidifier.

If you live in humid climates, then mold is always a concern, and you should have your house periodically checked by a professional. It's never a bad idea to add an air purifier to a bedroom, although they are never noise-free. One solution is to run them during the day and turn them off at night.

Another idea to consider is removing the carpeting from your bedroom. Most carpets tend to decrease air quality. Another is to make sure that your mattress and pillows are both non-toxic. Shop for non-toxic items the same way you shop for non-GMO products. Look for labels that say non-toxic.

If you have trouble sleeping, the first thing to eliminate is any stimulants from your diet, such as caffeine. You will feel tired at

Chapter Two: Rest

first and, perhaps, tired quite often. However, that tiredness will lead to more restful sleep. I often fall asleep within five minutes of when my head hits the pillow. A big reason is the lack of stimulants.

If you get run down from a lack of sleep, sleeping extra hours will help, but don't make this a habit. Constantly sleeping extra hours is probably a sign that you are not getting enough rest. For an extended life, you want to strive for a consistently rested body. The key, of course, is getting enough sleep on a nightly basis.

The next thing to help with sleeping is exercise. If you exercise vigorously, it will tire you out and help with sleep. I have found that exercise and sleep go hand in hand. They both help each other.

Another thing that is useful is reading. If you have trouble sleeping, turn off the TV or computer and read. Tire out your mind. If you find yourself reading a lot to fall asleep, then buy a light that has reduced blue spectrum. These are now easy to find. Just Google sleep lights.

Since I mentioned lights, it's probably a good idea for me to mention that LED lighting can impact sleep. LED lighting is primarily a blue light with an intensity that is about five times that found in nature. These intense blue lights are actually stimulating and can keep you from easily falling asleep. Exposing yourself to bright LED lights before bedtime is counter-productive to falling asleep. Conversely, they are great for waking up in the morning. The best light sources before bed are incandescent and halogen lights, or reduced blue spectrum LEDs.

A new bed is always a good idea to try for better sleep.

Sounds can help. Millions of people download various sounds that help induce sleep. In fact, there is a new product called Dreem that provides sounds that have been proven to induce sleep. It is sold by a company named Rythm that is based in San Francisco.

A strange sleep device is available, called Sense. It is sold by a company named Hello that is also based in San Francisco. The device will tell you what to change in your room to help you sleep better. It is a smart device that will answer your questions.

As you would expect, there are websites that want to help you with your sleep problem. Just Google sleep programs.

If you have tried all of the above and still have trouble sleeping, then you can try to use a supplement. There are three supplements which are useful for inducing sleep: Tryptophan, valerian root extract, and melatonin. All of these can be purchased at a vitamin supplement store. Since they are inexpensive, try all three and find out which one works best for you. Also, do a Google search and research each one.

Note that it is never a good practice to become dependent on a supplement for your nightly sleep. They should only be used on random occasions.

Chapter Three

TAKE SUPPLEMENTS

This chapter title should be named, *Take Supplements and Lots of Them*. Everyone should be taking handfuls of supplements on a daily basis. Why? Because our food quality is atrocious. Our soil has been depleted to the point that we have to eat large quantities to make up for the low nutritional content. We need to take supplements because it is impossible to eat large enough quantities of foods to get the nutrients we need.

Note: Vitamins and supplements are not risk free of side effects, and it is possible to overdose with some supplements. Make sure to research each vitamin and supplement that you take for side effects. And sure to use botanical supplements that were made from living plants and not synthetics made from chemicals.

While I implore you to take lots of supplements, I am not suggesting that you exceed a regular dosage of each. Many vitamins can be toxic and dangerous at high dosages. What I am suggesting is taking a wide variety of supplements on a daily basis.

For those of you who are skeptical about the effectiveness of supplements, I have learned that our bodies do, indeed, assimilate vitamins. If I take 100 milligrams of niacin, my body will literally heat up. If I take 500 milligrams, my face will turn red.

It is my non-professional opinion that a significant reason why nearly half of men and one-third of women will get cancer is because of a poor diet *and* a lack of supplements. By taking supplements and eating healthy, I believe that the risk of getting cancer is reduced substantially, perhaps even prevented. Moreover, it is a proven fact that many illnesses can be attributed to a mineral or vitamin deficiency.

If you eat healthily to boost your immune system and take supplements to prevent any mineral or vitamin deficiency, you have increased your odds of longevity. I've been taking supplements for over thirty years, and every year that passes I realize I should be taking more.

Because of soil depletion, it is nearly impossible to get enough vitamins and minerals from food sources alone. For this reason, you should be including a vitamin and mineral supplement in your daily routine. You can do this with multi-vitamin tablets. It's also a good idea to drink mineralized water, sometimes called colloidal minerals.

There have been many studies of communities where many members live until they are 100. One of the factors they usually find is highly mineralized water content from local springs. There is a likely correlation between life extension and the daily consumption of colloidal minerals.

The next supplement that is crucial for longevity is what are called antioxidants. Antioxidants can reduce free radicals which can induce premature aging. There are a myriad of antioxidants and they occur in most fruits, vegetables, herbs, tea, coffee, and nuts. However, you cannot get enough by eating food alone because you will have to eat large quantities. You want to consume an ORAC (oxygen radical absorbance capacity) value of 25,000 to 50,000 per day, which is nearly impossible without a supplement.

My antioxidant supplement has 42,000 ORAC in one pill. There are many different ones on the market.

Here is a partial list of common foods that have high ORAC values that you probably eat quite often:

Chapter Three: Take Supplements

Garlic, cinnamon, basil, parsley, rosemary, turmeric, ginger, blueberries, blackberries, raspberries, pomegranates, pistachios, almonds, lentils, black beans, pinto beans, artichokes, asparagus, and cranberries. It is a good idea to eat more of them.

Resveratrol is a good antioxidant supplement. It's also been known to increase energy in rats and mice, and perhaps even have anti-aging properties. Grape seed extract is similar to resveratrol and is also an excellent antioxidant.

I like to take vitamin C because it is both a strong antioxidant and an immune booster.

I like to take vitamin D and E because we are prone to deficiencies in both because of our poor food sources. If you plan to be outside in the sun, then you can skip your vitamin D supplement on that day. The human body can create its own vitamin D with sun exposure.

I take a cold-pressed flaxseed oil supplement that has omega-3, 6, and 9 fatty acids. I've read that the body can assimilate krill oil much easier that flaxseed oil, and it may be a superior supplement. Also, consider a cod liver oil supplement if you do not eat enough fish or raw nuts. Omega fatty acids are very good for the brain and blood vessels. I used to take fish oil, until the Fukushima disaster contaminated the ocean. If you consistently eat a lot of fish, such as salmon, then you probably do not need this supplement.

I am a vegetarian, so I take an iron supplement. An iron deficiency can cause tiredness and impact your blood and immune system. Leafy green vegetables are a good source of iron, but red meat is the best source. Unless you eat red meat, an iron supplement is not a bad idea.

As a vegetarian, I also take a plant-based protein powder supplement in a smoothie. Some vegetarians take these daily, but I only do it twice a week. I find that my regular diet has sufficient protein because I consume a lot of nuts, legumes, and peanut butter, plus my daily breakfast cereal has significant protein. If you consume meat, then it is unlikely that you will get a protein deficiency.

For anti-inflammation, turmeric, ginger, cinnamon, and pineapple are helpful.

For energy, resveratrol, vitamin B-12, ginkgo biloba, and ginseng are helpful.

For depression, niacin, lithium orotate, and raw cacao seeds are helpful.

I think that taking turmeric and cinnamon daily are perhaps the best supplements you can take. Both have powerful anti-inflammation properties.

If you have any pain in your body, then you probably also have inflammation. Try this each morning, Monday through Friday: mix one teaspoon of cinnamon with one tablespoon of raw, unfiltered honey. Consume it with an eight ounce glass of organic pineapple juice, along with two turmeric capsules. On weekends, drink lots of pure water.

To prevent inflammation, you can do this routine three days a week, with less of each ingredient: try one-half teaspoon of cinnamon, one teaspoon of raw, unfiltered, honey. Take with six ounces of organic pineapple juice, and one turmeric capsule.

The supplements I have listed should only be a starting point. Add whatever else that you think might help with your overall health. I have a few more that I take, but I have not listed them because I am not certain of their benefits. You too will likely try several different types. It's human nature to be curious. There are a myriad to choose from.

There are a few superfoods that you should include in your diet. I'll be talking about them in Chapter Five.

Chapter Four

REDUCE STRESS

There is a saying that stress is a killer. I agree with that. For this reason, you have to find ways to reduce stress. The ideal way is through a good marriage, which has been proven to increase your lifespan. If you don't have a good marriage, the next best way to reduce stress is through positive social interaction. If you are consistently laughing with your friends and family, then the odds are good that your stress levels are low.

If you don't have one of those factors in your life, then get a pet, preferably a dog or a cat. A good pet can reduce your stress levels almost as well as a fellow human. My cat purrs on my lap most days, and I talk to her frequently. From my perspective, we have a relationship that requires constant engagement. She might as well be a human because she has more emotion than some people I know. When I talk to her, she looks at me and I know that she understands. Often, when I won't let her be on my lap, she bites my feet. If that's not an expression of anger, I don't know what is. And you should see her eyes light up when I ask her if she wants to play hide and seek. Have you ever watched a cat run and hide? It's the funniest thing you ever saw, and it reduces stress like you would not believe.

So, those are the big three, but there are other things that you can do. Exercise is very good for reducing stress, and that is already on your agenda. Walking and hiking outside are also useful. Going to the movies or a concert helps. Attending conferences is a nice outlet, as are vacations. Hobbies are useful. Religion or spirituality helps. Reading is another stress remover. What do all of these things have in common? They are all relaxing.

The key to reducing stress is preventing it from reaching extreme levels. Stress causes cortisol to release from the adrenal glands. In chronic cases of stress, people release high levels of cortisol on a daily basis. This is really bad for longevity. Ideally, you want to limit the amount of cortisol that you release. Less is better.

You never know when stress is going to hit or how you will respond. I would think that everyone has felt its effects at some point in their life. My first experience was when I was in fifth grade and I was afraid of a bully, who was a couple of years older than me. I thought he was going to kill me. It was awful. In hindsight, he never laid a hand on me and the stress was self-created.

It turns out that nearly all stress is self-created. The exceptions are traumas that are usually not our fault, such as an accident. Stress is always fear run amok. It's a fear that won't leave you alone. It's a mindset that is the opposite of how you want to be. For longevity, you want to live with levity, joy, and peace of mind. That's the low-stress state that you want to strive to achieve.

To achieve a low-stress state of mind, you have to let go of willfulness. Instead of directing your life in a perpetual state of willfulness, you need to live with trust and surrender. This is somewhat counterintuitive to how we are taught to live. However, instead of trying to direct your life, accept what comes your way. Live with humility and gratitude. Most people are consumed with stress because they are always trying to control their lives. They refuse to let go and surrender. They always want to have a plan and to carry it out to the letter in a continual act of will.

How many people get stressed out because every detail in their life isn't going perfectly? This is from willfulness. Do you see how willfulness is stressful? Do you see how trying to control your life is stressful? Let go and surrender. Don't dwell on the past or worry about the future. Trust that it will work out. That's how you reduce stress. The more you can live in the now, the better off you will be from a longevity standpoint.

When I was about twenty years of age, I took a trip to Mexico with some friends. One of my friends had a beach house that his parents owned. While we were down there, I was mesmerized by these children who lived in a nearby house that had a dirt floor and no electricity. I had no idea that people in Mexico lived in such extreme poverty. What stunned me was their smiling faces. They were enjoying life more than we were. Now, how was that possible? We were on vacation, having the time of our lives. It was us that were supposed to be experiencing happiness, not them.

I thought about that experience for years before I figured it out. Those children were happy because they only cared about the present moment. They didn't care about their past or their future. They didn't care about what they didn't have, only about what was important, which was a loving family. They lived with humility and gratitude for what they had.

I still remember the smile on that ten-year-old boy's face. I was not as happy as he was, not even close. Why? Because I was trying to control my life. I was trying to create my own happiness. At that time, I had no idea that the secret to happiness is to let go and surrender. Once you stop forcing your will onto the future, you will be amazed at how stress becomes less of a factor in your life.

We need to become like that little boy who had nothing, but still felt like the happiest person on the planet. When you reach that same realization, stress will have a hard time finding you.

One method of obtaining this type of mindset is eliminating stuff that you do not need. Try to simplify your life. There are various strategies to obtain simplification. One is to toss out anything that you no longer use. Clean out your garage and storage areas with the intent of tossing out all non-essential items. Every few years, review your wardrobe and eliminate anything that you no longer intend to wear. Make it a proactive part of your life to continuously simplify your stuff.

Why simplification? Who do you think has more stress, someone with a myriad of stuff that they do not use, or someone who only keeps what he uses? Which one do you think has a better handle on their life? Can we measure someone's stress level by the cleanliness of their garage? Probably.

Another method to use is meditation. This is not easy to learn how to do, but it can be very effective. Perhaps the best time to meditate is when you wake up in the morning. If you quiet your mind for five or ten minutes, that can set the tone for the rest of the day.

So, use the various methods that I have given you to reduce stress, but more than that, find a way to keep stress out of your life. Stop worrying about the future and trying to control your life. Instead, trust that everything will work out for the best. Live with humility and gratitude. Count your blessings every day and put a smile on your face. If you can do that, then you will be amazed at how you can control your stress.

The key to reducing stress is keeping your mind out of the past and the future. Have you ever noticed that, when you are doing something that you enjoy, such as socializing with friends and family, that your mind is present? Or, if you are doing one of the activities that I listed, that your mind is present? When you are engaged in an activity, your mind is always present. This is why these activities are stress reducers. It's only when you start projecting into the future or dwelling on the past, that stress comes into being.

Chapter Four: Reduce Stress

Now that you know what triggers stress, you can try to keep your mind from running you ragged.

Let's end this chapter with a bit of levity. Two of the most joyful things that we do are both stress reducers and life extenders. They are laughter and sex. Studies show that people who laugh more and have more sex live longer. Makes sense to me. Hugh Hefner is ninety and still going strong. Coincidence? Probably not. Lol.

Chapter Five

EAT WELL

Disclaimer: This book includes advice on nutrition. However, I am a layman and have only learned through experience. If you are going to make any changes to your diet, then consultant with your physician.

* * * * *

The most difficult thing to do for good health is to eat well. For some people, it is impossible because of ingrained habits. It is probably the most formidable challenge you will face for improving your health. The irony is that once you change your eating habits, it becomes very easy to follow. The difficulty is in changing them.

Most of you are not going to like this chapter. That's because most of you are likely using food for satiation and not for health. If you want good health, then you will need to learn how to eat to live and to stop living to eat. There's a big difference. Ideally, everything that you consume should sustain good health. Once you achieve this attitude, the battle is won.

I didn't need to do very much research to write this chapter. I have been focusing on healthy eating for decades and I have learned quite a bit. If you take your nutrition seriously, then you will also be able to write this chapter, or something similar. Let's jump in and get started.

Eating well is all about exclusion and inclusion. You need to exclude certain foods and include others. Let's begin with what you need to exclude. Here is the list:

1) Refined sugar and sugar substitutes (except a few listed below).
2) Vegetable and plant-based oils (except a few listed below).
3) Simple carbohydrates (except infrequently).
4) Preservatives and additives (except infrequently).

You need to stop eating sugar on a regular basis, except for fruit and honey. Beet and cane sugar are not as bad as corn sugar, but they should all be avoided as much as possible. Moreover, all artificial sugar substitutes should be avoided. There are a few natural sugar substitutes, such as stevia and chicory, and it's okay to include some foods that include filtered cane sugar when done in low quantities or infrequently.

Why the exclusion of sugar? Because from a nutritional standpoint, it is clearly flawed and should be avoided as much as possible. It's like taking a drug. Sugar raises your blood sugar level, often quite dramatically, and puts stress on the body. The number one reason there is a diabetes epidemic is from the overconsumption of sugar. It's obvious that the body does not like it. In fact, some people consider sugar to be toxic.

A new book just came out called The Case Against Sugar. I haven't read it, but I did read some of the reviews. It's a diatribe against sugar. The story of sugar is steadily turning negative. In my opinion, the consumption of sugar is likely to decrease as more people become aware of its pitfalls.

If you exclude sugar from your diet, you will steadily come to realize that not only do you not need it, but you are glad you stopped eating it. It's kind of like stopping smoking. There is a relief that it is part of your past. This is a surefire sign that it is not good for you. In fact, it will become very difficult to eat pastries

Chapter Five: Eat Well

and other high sugar content foods. You will get used to saying, "No, thank you," when dessert is offered.

I do occasionally eat foods with sugar, such as at Christmas time. However, this is the rare occasion. I rarely bring sugary foods into my house, except, perhaps, some Italian cookies or banana bread given to me by a family member. On a yearly basis, these are rare events.

Many people are even more strict than me when it comes to sugar consumption. My advice is to be as strict as you can, without going crazy. Recognize sugar's flaws, but also recognize that a little bit won't make a difference to your overall health. It's okay to have dessert once in a while.

Next, exclude vegetable and plant-based oils from your regular diet. The only oils that are healthy are avocado, coconut, and cold-pressed extra-virgin olive oil. Some people even consider olive oil to be unhealthy, but not me. Although, do not heat up olive oil, and only eat it at room temperature. If you need to cook with heated oil, use coconut oil if possible, or else canola oil. I occasionally eat with heated canola oil, such as to make taco shells, but it is on an infrequent basis.

Note: There are different thoughts on using olive oil or avocado oil for frying. Do your own research. Many researchers think that they are safe for frying.

Without vegetable and plant-based oils in your regular diet, this means you can only eat fried foods on rare occasions. You may find that some of the foods you are currently consuming on a regular basis have these oils. I suggest that they be removed from your diet, or reduced to an infrequent basis. I still eat french fries, but only a few times a year.

Both olive oil and avocado oil are mono-unsaturated oils. This makes them healthy to consume at room temperature (in

29

my opinion). Coconut oil is saturated, but has unique properties, making it less susceptible to causing cardiovascular damage, even when heated during cooking. Coconut oil consumed at room temperature is perhaps the healthiest oil. I consider raw coconut to be a superfood, and highly beneficial to the body.

Most vegetable and plant-based oils can create plaque buildup in our arteries, which can lead to heart disease. When vegetable oil is heated, it creates oxidation, which is known to create adverse effects in the body. These are the main culprits for the thousands of heart surgeries that occur in this country. And it's not just fried foods to worry about. Hydrogenated oils, also called trans-fats, are in myriads of processed foods. These can be just as harmful as fried foods.

Whenever you read a food label and see the word oil, you can bet that it is not one of the three good oils that I have listed for regular consumption. More likely, you will see one of the vegetable or plant-based oils listed, or the term, hydrogenated oil. You want to avoid these as much as possible.

The next thing to avoid is simple carbohydrates. These are what many people call comfort foods, such as snacks, chips, pastries, and desserts. Just about every snack or dessert is made from simple carbohydrates – anything that is processed, such as chips, crackers, bread, candy, cereal (nearly all), pastries, pies, cakes, cookies, and soda pop. None of these foods is very nutritious because they are made from processed simple carbs, which generally have low nutrient levels. To make matters worse, they are immediately converted by the process of digestion into blood sugar (glucose) and, often, into fat – if you already have too much sugar in your system. The immediate conversion into blood sugar is why these are the feel-good foods. You can also call them the temptation foods. As I said earlier, sugar is like taking a drug.

Chapter Five: Eat Well

Most foods now are labeled with a carbohydrate count. If you read the labels of the foods I listed as simple carbs, you will see that they all have a high carbohydrate count. This is why they can make you fat fairly quickly. Anytime you consume more than approximately 30 grams of carbs at one meal, there is the potential for your blood sugar level to get overloaded. Once you overload, your pancreas will secrete extra insulin to lower the amount of sugar in your blood. The excess sugar goes to the liver, which will create fat from the excess sugar. Basically, your body tells your liver that it has plenty of sugar for energy, and to go ahead and create some fat, in case it needs energy later.

Note: It is difficult to eat a meal with less than 30 grams of carbohydrates. Most of my meals are 50 to 60 grams of carbohydrates. I weigh 150 lbs., so adjust accordingly. I have found this is the right amount of carbohydrates for me. The only reason to stay under 30 is if you are trying to lose weight or to ensure that you do not gain weight.

Now you know where nearly all of our fat comes from: the overconsumption of carbohydrates. If you consume less than 30 grams of carbohydrates for a meal, it is nearly impossible for the body to generate excess fat, although you could do it by consuming large quantities of meat or, perhaps, cheese. How people normally gain weight is from overconsuming carbohydrates, and simple carbohydrates are usually the culprits.

So, simple carbs are bad in two ways. First, they have very little nutritious content. Second, once you overload your body with too much sugar, you generate fat.

It's not bad for you to consume simple carbs once in a while. The key is to do it at infrequent times and to not go overboard. Sure, it won't be nutritious, but you will enjoy it, and I suppose it is an energy source, even though it is comprised of mostly empty calories. A little bit of popcorn at the cinema won't stop your quest for a healthy life, but try to keep it out of your pantry. In fact, it would be a good idea to keep your pantry as bare as possible of simple carbs and processed foods. I have learned that if you keep comfort food in your house, it will get eaten.

The next thing to avoid is preservatives and additives. These are mostly chemicals and not food. When you read a label and don't know what the listed ingredient is, you can bet that it is a preservative or additive. An additive is supposed to make the food either look better or taste better. The worst additive is probably MSG (monosodium glutamate), which the food industry loves, and I detest. It adds flavoring and shelf life, but has several potential negative side effects. It's amazing that this stuff is legal. Google it and find out for yourself.

If MSG is legal, then what other preservatives and additives are we ingesting with our processed foods that are unhealthy? I think we have to assume the worst and avoid them as much as possible. If you are not a label reader, it's time to start.

After you begin reading labels, preservatives and additives will become obvious because they do not sound like natural foods. Sometimes, you will find labels with literally dozens of words that you cannot pronounce. Any food ingredient that you have never heard of, or can't pronounce, is likely to be a preservative or an additive.

Some preservatives to avoid are sulfites, nitrates, BHA, BHT, bromate, and sulfur. These preservatives usually appear as longer words, such as sodium nitrate, sodium sulfite, sodium benzoate, or sulfur dioxide. Anything that has one of these words is suspicious, at best.

Are there any healthy preservatives or additives that the food industry uses? Perhaps, pectin, which is made from fruit, but I'm not aware of any others. And don't trust foods just because they

Chapter Five: Eat Well

are sold at a health food store, or have an organic label. Many of these foods still contain unhealthy preservatives or additives. Read all labels.

One category not on my exclusion list that many people exclude is some dairy products. There have been studies that indicate that dairy products may cause inflammation, but these studies are not definitive and people react differently. Milk does have a protein called casein that is very similar to gluten in molecular structure. I have switched from using cow's milk to almond milk because I know that almond milk is healthy, and I'm not sure about cow's milk. I've read that many cows are given pharmaceutical drugs and hormones to keep them from getting sick and to increase their milk production. Plus, I'm not ecstatic about how cows are milked by machines in cramped quarters.

Note: Butter has a negligible amount of casein because butter contains very little protein. Also, butter made from grass-fed cows is actually one of the few healthy saturated fats. I wouldn't cook with butter, but eating it at room temperature is fine.

My suggestion is to use dairy in moderation, and it won't curtail your health. I personally would not eat cheese or any other dairy product daily, but I'm not convinced that dairy is bad for everyone. Keep it moderate and infrequent. Pizza a few times a year will not hurt your overall health.

Simple carbs are much worse for you than a little bit of dairy. Where dairy becomes a problem is when you are already consuming a lot of meat, then you tend to get too much cholesterol. Also, many people are lactose intolerant or sensitive to casein. But for the rest of us, we can eat a little bit of butter, cheese, and eggs from time to time (note that eggs are not a dairy product).

Note: There is no reason to consume cholesterol because the body can create what it needs. Cholesterol is only found in animal products and those on a vegan diet (which is free of animal products) have been tested for low cholesterol levels. Vegans have been found to have sufficient cholesterol levels.

Another food that is excluded by many is gluten, which generally is associated with wheat products, although it also is found in barley, rye, and malt (unless it is fermented). Gluten is considered to create inflammation. I personally eat wheat on occasion, and consider gluten intolerance to be genetic, and not incurred by everyone. However, it is not a bad idea to limit your gluten exposure. Since I eat a lot of pasta, I have switched to gluten-free pasta, although I'm probably wasting my time. If pasta was unhealthy for everyone, we would know. I'm half Italian and I've known a lot of Italians who have eaten pasta all of their life. Unless you have a known gluten intolerance, I have my doubts it is unhealthy.

For men (and possibly women), exclude unfermented soy. The reason why is because unfermented soy contains estrogen-like isoflavones. For this reason, consuming too much soy can lower men's testosterone levels. If you are a woman, this shouldn't be a problem, although some research seems to indicate that unfermented soy is unhealthy for either sex. But for a man, estrogen is something better to be avoided.

When you dine out, try to avoid fried foods, as well as white and butter sauces. Many of these sauces contain MSG and hydrogenated oils. They will taste great, but your body won't like them. For this reason, try to eat out as little as possible.

* * * * *

Now we get to discuss what to include in your diet. Here is the list:

Chapter Five: Eat Well

1) Vegetables.
2) Fruits.
3) Complex carbohydrates.
4) Nuts.
5) Legumes and whole grains.
6) Superfoods.
7) Unsaturated and saturated fats.
8) Meat (optional).

Vegetables are probably the most important food source for a healthy life. The reason why is because they have an abundance of vitamins and minerals that keep you healthy. In fact, vegetables are the best anti-cancer food source (fruits and some teas are a close second). If you are going to consistently obtain nutritional requirements for good health, then vegetables will be required.

Ideally, you want to eat vegetables every day, and don't be afraid to have large portions. I normally eat three vegetables with dinner. Most people would think I eat too many green beans or too much kale with dinner, but I believe that the nutritional content has diminished over the years. We now have to eat more to get the same nutrition that previous generations received.

Ideally, you want to eat vegetables raw. However, this is not always possible. For instance, I do not like green beans, broccoli, or asparagus raw and have to steam them. You want to be careful with what you put on vegetables, which I covered previously on which foods to exclude from your diet.

Experiment with different vegetables. Over the years, I have tried many different kinds to find which ones I like the best. Everyone has different taste preferences, and your taste will change over time. You will be surprised how your taste changes once you begin to eat more vegetables and exclude non-nutritious foods.

If you find that you simply do not like vegetables, then you can juice them and combine them with fruit to improve the flavor. This is an ideal way to include them in your diet because juicing can include raw vegetables.

Here is my list of preferred vegetables:

1) Broccoli.
2) Asparagus.
3) Leafy greens (green leaf, romaine, kale, chard, beetroot leaf, spinach, parsley).
4) Green beans.
5) Carrots.
6) Celery.
7) Radishes.
8) Tomatoes.
9) Red and white onions.
10) Beetroot.
11) Zucchini.
12) Brussel sprouts.
13) Cabbage.
14) Green and red bell peppers.
15) Artichokes.
16) Mushrooms.
17) Olives.
18) Cucumber.
19) Shallots.
20) Cauliflower.

Chapter Five: Eat Well

* * * * *

The next food source of importance is fruit. Fruits are important because of their antioxidant properties and ability to neutralize free-radicals. Fruits are also nutritious and help boost the immune system. I try to eat some type of fruit every day and most days, I eat two or three different fruits. Do not consume mass quantities of fruit during a single meal because they are high in sugar. A single apple or a single orange is sufficient. A few slices of melon or a couple of handfuls of grapes is plenty for a single serving.

Here is my list of preferred fruits:

1) Apple.
2) Pineapple.
3) Grapefruit.
4) Lemon.
5) Grapes.
6) Melon (cantaloupe, watermelon, honeydew).
7) Dark berries (blueberry, strawberry, blackberry, raspberry).
8) Avocado.
9) Plums.
10) Cherries.
11) Peach.
12) Pear.
13) Orange, tangerine, tangelo.
14) Banana.
15) Apricot.
16) Kiwi.
17) Figs.

18) Mango.

19) Pomegranate.

20) Papaya.

It is okay to replace fresh vegetables or fresh fruit with a frozen source. It turns out that very little nutrition is lost from freezing.

Let's review, so that you have this understood. Every day you need to eat both fruits and vegetables. These are now a daily requirement. You will find that your lifestyle begins to change just from that single decision. You will begin to eat healthily, and you will plan to eat healthily. Plans become habits, and habits become lifestyles.

It's not easy to eat healthily because it requires a lifestyle change. You will find that habits are hard to break. I recommend starting with fruits and vegetables. Once you have your daily habit down of including fruits and vegetables into your diet, the rest of your diet will be easier to change.

* * * * *

The third item to include in your diet is complex carbohydrates. These are the good carbohydrates when consumed in moderation. They include pasta, rice, potatoes, and oats. These are the carbohydrates that do not spike your blood sugar the way that simple carbohydrates do. Instead, the body stores these energy sources in an efficient manner, and then disburses it slowly over a period of hours. This is why marathon runners fill up on these food sources the night before a race.

When you eat complex carbohydrates for dinner, that energy source is available the next day. It is, by far, the most efficient energy source the body uses. The only thing you need to remember about complex carbohydrates is that if you overconsume the number

Chapter Five: Eat Well

of grams of carbohydrates, then the pancreas releases too much insulin, and the liver can turn the excess carbs into fat. For this reason, it is smart to consume small portions.

I used to eat large portions of pasta or rice. Now I only consume about 30 or 40 grams of carbohydrates per meal, which is actually a small portion. This is about the optimal amount to avoid putting stress on the pancreas and avoiding fat creation. It is nearly impossible to generate fat if you keep your carbohydrate intake low.

If you are exercising intensely, you can double your complex carbohydrate consumption and not gain fat. The body is smart enough to "carb load" and not generate fat. The body knows that you plan to use this energy in the near term. Cyclists and long-distance runners consume large quantities of complex carbs and remain thin as a rail.

While potatoes are good carbohydrates, I consider them inferior to rice and pasta. First of all, rice and pasta are easy to cook, which makes it conducive to including them in your daily diet. Second, potatoes are part of the nightshade family (sweet potatoes are not), which are known to cause inflammation in some people. Potatoes can have the same issue as gluten and induce inflammation.

It's okay to eat potatoes, just do it on an infrequent basis. While not all people are affected by inflammation, it's still a possibility. Also, potatoes tend to be cooked in oil or butter. I do like baked potatoes on occasion, and I find that the skin is delicious. If you are at a restaurant and want to find something healthy to eat, a good choice is a baked potato and a salad.

I'm probably being too harsh on potatoes. They are an ideal energy source, plus they are high in iodine, which is necessary for a healthy thyroid. In fact, thyroid hormones are important for our energy levels. There are not many food sources that are high in iodine; the other common ones are navy beans and strawberries. If you do not eat a lot of potatoes, then try to consume strawberries on a consistent basis. You can also get iodine from iodized salt, which is salt that has had an iodine additive.

For complex carbohydrates, I prefer gluten-free pasta, although I also eat brown rice. My preferred gluten-free kinds of pasta are made out of brown rice, lentils, quinoa, or chickpeas. I do occasionally eat regular wheat pasta when I eat out or at a family dinner.

Some of the longest living people are from Asia, where white rice is their daily staple. The other thing that they consistently include in their daily diet is a variety of vegetables. While I do not include rice on my superfood list, it is perhaps the best and most efficient source of energy. If there is a perfect food, it's probably rice. If I were Asian, I'm sure I would eat more rice than pasta.

My ideal serving size for rice is one-quarter cup uncooked, which is 40 grams of carbohydrates. For pasta, my ideal serving size is one-half cup of uncooked pasta, which contains 38 grams of carbs. It took me a while to adjust to these lower portions. At first, it will feel like you are not eating enough. However, if you are eating complex carbohydrates daily, you will find that is enough to give you energy.

I am five feet, ten inches tall and weigh 160 lbs., so adjust your portions accordingly. I have learned from experience that one-third of a cup of uncooked rice and three-fourths of a cup of uncooked pasta is too much, and I end up feeling too full after eating. Try to learn your ideal portions and consistently use them. Your body is smart enough to remember how to handle your portions.

Some nutritionists consider white rice to be empty calories because, other than energy, it does not contain a lot of vitamins. However, it is an excellent source of energy. Brown rice includes bran, which has significant levels of manganese and fiber, making it a more nutritious choice. However, you do not want to eat brown rice every day because it contains small amounts of arsenic and phytic acid (more about this below). I only eat brown rice twice a week. If you want to eat rice more than twice a week, then eat white rice. An important fact about rice is that it can go bad within 30 days if it is exposed to air. For this reason, store your rice in an airtight container.

Occasionally, I will eat one cup of uncooked pasta or more, but these are exceptions when I am eating out (or family meals), and the quality of food is exceptional. These rare splurges are not going to hurt your overall health, but don't make it a habit. Note that I always feel afterward like I overate, with a very full stomach. This is another reason to make your own meals as often as possible. You are less likely to overconsume when you cook at home.

Oats, a highly nutritious and quality energy source, are probably the most ignored complex carbohydrate, although some people eat oatmeal for breakfast. But for the most part, few people eat oats consistently.

If you dislike hot oatmeal, it's easy to make your own cold oat cereal. Combine raw rolled oats, raw chopped almonds, raw sunflower seeds, and raisins (or dried cranberries). Eat it with unsweetened almond milk and blueberries.

Note: Oats need to be soaked in liquid before eating. Do not eat them dry.

Note: If you eat your cereal with almond milk, I have found that you only need about three ounces of almond milk and the rest water. This gives it the same density as non-fat milk and the flavor is fine. Also, when you mix your almond milk with water it costs half the price.

One of the benefits of eating oats is that it will lower your bad LDL cholesterol levels. There are not many foods that will directly lower your LDL cholesterol. The two most common ones are oats and beans.

You do not need to include complex carbohydrates in your diet every day, but it is a good idea to include them several times a week. Why? Because they will keep you energized, and they are ideal for maintaining your weight. Complex carbohydrates will make you feel full and you are less likely to snack. I rarely snack and the reason why is because I normally consume complex carbohydrates for breakfast and dinner.

If I have a salad for dinner that excludes complex carbs, I can often tell that I skipped my complex carbs if I exercise the following day. Try to keep your body loaded with complex carbs to keep your energy levels high.

Here is my list of preferred complex carbohydrates:

1) Pasta.
2) Rice.
3) Oats.
4) Russet and red potatoes.
5) Sweet potatoes.

* * * * *

The next category is nuts. I would say fewer people eat raw nuts regularly than exercise regularly. Very few people grasp the nutritional value of nuts. Edgar Cayce, who was called the sleeping prophet, said that eating two or three almonds every day was an excellent way to ensure good health. He even called almonds vitamins.

People think that nuts are fattening. That's a myth. I usually eat nuts daily and I'm thin. People will eat simple carbs, which are

Chapter Five: Eat Well

fattening, and then skip nuts. As long as you only eat a handful of nuts per serving, you won't gain weight. The key to nut consumption is moderation. The handful rule works extremely well.

I do have one caveat to my handful rule. If you consume your normal amount of calories and then eat an additional handful of nuts for dessert every day, then you will gain weight. In other words, if you overconsume nuts, it is easy to gain weight. However, do not be afraid of gaining weight by consuming nuts as part of your normal diet.

Nuts are very nutritious, and they contain healthy omega-3 and 6 polyunsaturated fatty acids. I find it interesting that nutrition begins with the word nut. Someone is trying to tell us something. Consuming nuts raw is the best way to eat them because they have a higher nutritional content than processed or roasted nuts.

I prefer raw almonds and walnuts, but I eat a lot of different types from time to time. Have you noticed that walnuts are shaped like the brain? Do you think this is a coincidence? Not likely. Mother Nature is trying to tell us something. Also, almonds are actually not a nut. They are seeds. Perhaps this is why they have such a high nutritional value.

Try to eat nuts on a daily basis – one handful a day. A daily basis isn't a requirement, but try to make it a habit of eating raw nuts multiple times per week. Nuts are expensive. For this reason, you have to tell yourself that they are required in your diet. The cheapest form is peanut butter, although peanuts are actually a legume, not a nut. Most other nuts are not cheap. When I go to Trader Joe's, I tend to spend more than I want to on nuts.

Here is my list of preferred nuts/seeds:

1) Raw almonds (seeds).
2) Raw walnuts.
3) Chia seeds (soak first).

4) Pistachios.
5) Raw sunflower seeds.
6) Raw brazil nuts.
7) Raw macadamia nuts.
8) Raw cacao nuts (seeds).
9) Raw pecans.
10) Hazel nuts.

Are you starting to catch on? You want to consume nutritious food and exclude non-nutritious food. If you exclude nuts from your regular diet, you are depriving yourself of an excellent source of nutrition. As Edgar Cayce said, if you want to be healthy, eat more almonds.

I did not include cashews on my list because of the way so many come to the market. Most cashews are grown in poor countries and workers are subjected to less than favorable working conditions. The reason why is because the shell of a cashew is poisonous on the outside and toxic on the inside! It is dangerous to process and must be done in a careful manner. As you can imagine, workers are not exactly a high priority in some of these countries. There are many ugly stories about what is happening. In India, many cashew workers went on strike to improve working conditions to alleviate the exposure to poisons and toxins. Many people call them blood cashews because of this situation. Until this labor issue is fixed, I have stopped eating them.

In the USA, it can be difficult to find raw, unpasteurized nuts in retail stores. The packaging may say raw, but they probably aren't. Instead, they are likely pasteurized using either steam or fumigation. These processes may kill bacteria, but also reduce the nutritional content.

In California, where nearly all USA almonds and walnuts are produced, all nuts to be sold as raw are pasteurized. In fact, it is illegal for retail stores in California to sell raw, unpasteurized nuts. Yet, most packaging lists the nuts as raw. Currently, as of 2018, a nut label does not have to say if it was pasteurized. In California (and many other states), if you want raw, unpasteurized nuts, then you have to buy them online and they are imported. As you can imagine, raw, imported almonds are expensive.

* * * * *

Next is legumes and whole grains. Legumes are beans. A lot of people do not like beans because they cause gas. However, not eating beans is a mistake. As long as you keep your portions small, you should get very little gas. Moreover, it is usually the foods that you consume with beans that cause gas, such as meat. Try to eat a salad for a meal that contains beans and see if you get any gas.

Note: Raw legumes, grains, and brown rice should all be soaked before cooking. This is required to reduce the phytic acid they contain, which can lead to mineral deficiencies. I won't go into soaking methods, but please do some research if you cook these raw foods.

Pinto beans, black beans, kidney beans, navy beans, and lentils are all highly nutritious. They include significant quantities of fiber, vitamins, minerals, and protein. Also, beans are one of the few foods that lower bad LDL cholesterol. You don't need to eat these on a daily basis, although you can. The key is to include them in your diet on a regular basis.

Here is my list of preferred legumes:
1) Pinto beans.
2) Black beans.
3) Peanuts.
4) Peas.

5) Garbanzo beans (chickpeas).

6) Lentils.

7) Kidney beans.

8) Navy beans.

Peas and peanuts are legumes, but I have a hard time not considering peas to also be a vegetable and peanuts to also be a nut. This is why peas have a high protein content, and why peanuts are inexpensive. The best powdered protein, in my opinion, is made from peas. Ironically, they call these vegetable protein powders. I buy vegetable protein powder, and the first ingredient is always peas, which is not a vegetable!

I like unsweetened peanut butter. "Adams" brand unsweetened creamy peanut butter is unbelievably good. Most people do not recognize the nutritional value of peanut butter. I like to eat it with celery, but it is also good on a sandwich. Peanut butter and jelly with real fruit spread is a healthy combination. Just make sure to go sugar-free and on whole grain bread.

Whole grains are not necessarily a requirement for a regular diet, but they are acceptable. The one thing to be cognizant of is that whole grains are nutritious. In fact, they can be as nutritious as nuts. Often, they include gluten, but not always. Whole grain non-gluten bread or pancakes can be a good addition to your regular diet. My favorite sandwich is almond butter and Smucker's strawberry real fruit spread on Ezekiel sprouted whole grain bread.

I eat Grape-nuts, which is a whole grain cereal. There are many whole grain cereals on the market, and they make an excellent breakfast. I have eaten Grape-nuts for years. Amazingly, it has 45 grams of complex carbohydrate in only a half cup. So, you need to consume small portions. I usually add raisins and sometimes blueberries, which brings it to 55 to 65 grams of carbohydrates.

Chapter Five: Eat Well

That's a high carbohydrate count for a daily meal, but it's the first meal of the day and the body is craving food. That's not a bad time to push the limits. I usually can go six to eight hours before I get hungry after this type of breakfast. In fact, I'm rarely hungry after five hours. That shows you how the body likes whole grains and complex carbs.

I get the same response from my body when eating oats for breakfast that I do with whole grains. However, oats have a lower carbohydrate count. There are 29 grams of carbohydrate in a half cup of raw rolled oats. By the way, it's okay to eat raw rolled oats as long as you soak them in a liquid, such as almond milk, before consumption. Most people soak them in hot water to make oatmeal.

* * * * *

Superfoods should be included in your diet because they offer enormous boosts to the immune system and overall health. In actuality, there is no such thing as a superfood. However, over time, more and more people have recognized that certain foods have special nutritional qualities. Thus, they have been deemed to be superfoods. Of course, there is no definitive list of which ones are superfoods, and I'm sure there are scholars who would question some of the foods on my list.

Here is a list of my preferred superfoods:
1) Lemon.
2) Turmeric.
3) Garlic.
4) Ginger.
5) Dark berries (goji, acai, blackberries, pomegranate, blueberries, raspberries).
6) Flax and chia seeds.

7) Green tea, Rooibos tea.
8) Raw cacao nuts.
9) Maca powder.
10) Spirulina and chlorella powder.
11) Beetroot.
12) Avocado.
13) Wild Salmon.
14) Coconut.
15) Almonds.
16) Hemp hearts.
17) Cinnamon.
18) Kelp and seaweed.

There are certain foods that are just amazingly nutritious. All of the foods listed above can be included in that category. Turmeric, garlic, and ginger are all very good at reducing inflammation (as is pineapple). Lemon is a magical fruit that helps the body to become pH neutral. It has an alkalizing ability to reduce acidic levels. No other fruit can do this, which I find fascinating. It also is known to detox the body and reduce inflammation.

Dark-colored berries contain polyphenols which have strong antioxidant properties that fight free radicals. They also can reverse cardiovascular disease. One man had nearly total blockage of his arteries. After several months of eating large quantities of dark berries, his blockages were down to sixty percent. He had bypass surgery and the berries saved his life. Just think how good they are at preventing cardiovascular disease.

Flax and chia seeds are like nuts on steroids, as far as nutritional content. Other nuts with high nutritional content are walnuts, brazil nuts, and pistachios.

Green tea and rooibos tea are high antioxidant drinks.

Chapter Five: Eat Well

Cacao nuts are processed into cocoa powder, which is made into chocolate. Raw cacao nuts have a high magnesium content and are very nutritious. They also have high antioxidant properties. The stimulant that gives you a high when you eat chocolate is called theobromine. This why cacao is called the food of the gods. Some people say that theobromine is the closest thing that replicates the feeling after you have sex. What's amazing is that theobromine is only found in cacao nuts.

Mother Nature did not want people to go crazy eating raw cacao nuts, so she made them toxic to the liver in high dosages. It is recommended that you only eat, at most, five or ten raw cacao nuts a day. To make chocolate, cacao nuts are roasted to remove the toxicity. This also reduces the level of theobromine and nutrition content. However, if you put fifteen or twenty raw cacao nuts in a blender with a frozen banana and eight ounces of water, you will have a tasty chocolate flavored happy drink that lasts for hours. I recommend only drinking this once or twice a week, as it can be addictive and toxic to the liver if over-consumed.

You can also include niacin, lithium orotate, ginseng, and vitamin B-12 to ensure that you have an energetic happy drink. However, based on my experience, the raw cacao nuts usually do the trick by themselves. You can experiment with some of these ingredients and find out what works for you.

Spirulina and chlorella are perhaps the most densely nutritious foods on the planet. They are both green powders that come from algae. You can literally live off these, which is unbelievable, but true. If you mix these with water, it is enough nutrition to stay alive. How is that for a highly nutritious food source? They are excellent additions for green smoothies.

Beetroot is another nutrition-packed food source. Some people call these beets. They are the hard, reddish-purple vegetables that you see in the produce section of the grocery store, usually chilled.

They sometimes have their leaves attached, which is another highly nutritious food source that can be juiced.

The best way to consume most of these superfoods is through juicing or smoothies. Find a way to get as many of these as possible into your regular diet.

* * * * *

Unsaturated and saturated fats are both required by the body, especially the brain, which is made of mostly fat. You want to consume the majority of your fat through unsaturated oils. These include cold-pressed extra virgin olive oil, avocados, nuts, and seeds. For saturated oil, you can use coconut oil or canola oil. Other sources include quality butter (grass-fed if possible), cheese, or egg yolks. As I mentioned earlier, the best way to consume oil is at room temperature and not heated. This also applies to butter, which can be considered an oil.

In case you were not aware, margarine is not butter or even a dairy product. It is made from hydrogenated vegetable oil. For this reason, I would not consider it a substitute for real butter.

If you consume meat, then obtaining saturated fat is not an issue. Animal sources are loaded with saturated fats. Another place to get saturated fat is vegetable oil. This is prevalent in the standard American diet and should be avoided as much as possible.

* * * * *

The last required food source is meat. Of course, this does not apply if you are a vegetarian or vegan. Some people prefer a vegetarian or vegan diet, and others do not. I think this has a lot to do with our blood type and genetics. My blood type is A+,

Chapter Five: Eat Well

which is very conducive to being a vegetarian. I personally feel healthy as a vegetarian and do not crave meat. If you try to become a vegetarian and you feel awful, then it is probably not something your body is ready for at this time, or if ever.

Note: Type A blood types (35% of the population) find it the easiest to be a vegetarian. Type O blood types (45% of the population) are usually meat eaters. And type B (10% of the population) or other rare blood types, have a better chance of being a vegetarian than Type O. Find out your blood type. If you have type A, then you might want to give vegetarian or vegan a try. Also, if you have a child that doesn't like meat, it might be normal if they have type A blood.

I have known many people who have tried to become a vegetarian, but went back to eating meat. I'll bet many of them had type O blood. Most people who experiment with being a vegetarian end up making some type of dietary change with their meat consumption. Some people end up eating more fish and less red meat, or more chicken and less red meat, but some type of new approach usually results.

If you include meat in your diet, now is the time to reduce its regularity. There is no reason to eat meat on a daily basis, from a nutrition standpoint. The nutritional content of meat is not high enough to be a daily requirement. First of all, meat is not a good energy source, although it is a good source of vitamins, minerals, protein, and iron.

The problem with meat is that it is difficult to digest, especially red meat. By eating meat on a daily basis, you are putting undue stress on your digestive system. Red meat can takes days to go through your system, whereas fruit and vegetables can go through in less than 24 hours. Meat acts like a blocker, blocking the path of other foods trying to get through. Do you see how this is not the most optimal way to eat?

There are two other inherent weaknesses with meat. First, it is high in saturated fat. Yes, the body needs saturated fat, but not a lot. Second, it is high in cholesterol. Thus, a high meat-based diet can result in high bad cholesterol (LDL).

If you like meat, then there is no problem consuming it a few times a week, just don't make it a daily habit. The more meat you consume, especially red meat, the more stress you are putting on your digestive system. Sure, the body is an amazing machine and can handle the stress, but you are reducing the likelihood of good health. In fact, you are increasing the likelihood of illness. I was reading recently how a study linked constipation with an array of illnesses. Once you reduce meat from your diet, bowel movements should become much more frequent and consistent.

If you feel that meat is something that you need to have in your diet, then I would suggest fish. The body can digest small amounts of fish much more efficiently than other forms of meat. Plus, fish has omega-3, 6, and 9 fatty acids that are highly nutritious.

The potential for colon cancer has literally exploded in the last few decades. The best way to reduce your risk of colon cancer is to reduce your meat consumption and increase your consumption of vegetables, fruits, nuts, legumes, whole grains, and superfoods. It is my opinion that the best cancer fighter is to live a lifestyle that proactively seeks healthy choices.

There are several replacement foods for meat. Some of these are eaten in pairs to create a complete protein. These pairs include rice and beans, pasta and peas, whole grain bread and peanut butter, hummus and whole wheat pita bread, spirulina and nuts or seeds. In addition to these pairs, some foods are complete proteins, such as soy, quinoa, buckwheat, chia seeds, and Ezekiel bread.

Here are some examples of meals that exclude meat and provide a source of protein. The combination of rice and beans is one of

Chapter Five: Eat Well

my favorite meals and is an excellent way to get protein. One of the reasons for quinoa's popularity is its protein potency. Making protein-rich buckwheat pancakes results in an extremely healthy breakfast. Adding chia seeds or spirulina to a smoothie makes an ideal protein drink. A peanut butter sandwich on Ezekiel bread is another potent protein food combination.

* * * * *

Here are a few notes for your diet.

Try to eat less, with smaller portions. Recognize that you are probably eating too much at each meal.

Try to limit your processed food intake. When you go to the grocery store, the vast majority of the food you purchase should not be processed. When you checkout at the grocery store, look at your items and see how many are processed. If it is more than ten percent, then you need to make some changes.

Do not snack. Instead, eat three meals a day and try not to skip meals. You could eat four or five smaller meals if that fits your dietary habits. When you consume smaller meals, it is much easier on your digestive system. I personally prefer three meals a day, plus a dessert of fruit and nuts eaten at least an hour after dinner.

Limit your intake of corn. Most corn (ninety percent or more) sold in the US is now a GMO variety. Also, any processed corn is a starch and a simple carbohydrate.

Limit your intake of chemicals and pesticides. Many people today try to avoid non-organic fruits and vegetables. The main reason why is because most fruits and vegetables are sprayed with pesticides. This is not allowed on organic food. Also, organic food is always non-GMO.

Do not use a microwave. The Russian studies on microwaves are not confidence boosting. Did you know that, if you put blood in a microwave and then inject it into someone, that they will die? Or, that, if you water a plant using microwaved water, the plant will die? The microscopic pictures of frozen water crystals after being microwaved is also unnerving. Google it. If water looks that ugly, what is happening to the food we microwave?

Do not cook with aluminum pans. There is some evidence that high aluminum levels in the brain correlate to Alzheimer's and dementia. This is another reason not to eat out often.

When eating out, be wary of preservatives, additives, GMOs, and hydrogenated oils.

Try to avoid fast food, if possible, which sometimes can't be avoided. If you are forced to eat fast food, a salad or a baked potato is always a good choice. A veggie bowl with rice at Chipotle is a good choice or, perhaps, a veggie sub from Subway. There aren't a lot of good choices out there for fast food.

Chapter Six

Drink Well

For some of you, you are going to have to increase your water consumption. Water is the body's cleaner. It cleans out the stomach and intestines. However, it is even more important than that. An amazing fifty to sixty percent of the body is made of water! Cells are actually seventy percent water. We think we are full of blood. No, it's water.

You probably know that the body is constantly rebuilding itself. For instance, cells never last very long. Instead, they are regenerated. Well, all of the water in our body needs to be constantly replaced. For this reason, we should consume mostly water. It should not only be our liquid of choice, but our priority.

How much water are you going consume on a daily basis, and what is the quality of that water? Well, if you are going to pursue life extension, then it better be about 32 ounces of water, and double that would be acceptable. And make sure your water is as pure as possible.

Tap water is nearly always low quality. If it has a bad taste, you can be certain the quality is low. I recommend getting a Zerowater water tester. They are about $20, but very valuable. You can get one on Amazon.com. You can test bottled water, tap water, even restaurant water. Most restaurants, including soda fountains, use filters to avoid a bad taste. For this reason, tap water at most restaurants is usually just as good as bottled water.

Fruits and vegetables have water content, but this is not part of your 32-ounce minimum. You need to consume a lot of pure water to flush out your system and keep it humming like a top.

You need to keep your body efficient in order to put less stress on it and keep your immune system boosted. Water is the ingredient that keeps everything in working order. Food adds nutrients, but water puts them to work. Water keeps your digestive system clean and in tip-top shape.

When I had my first colonoscopy at age fifty-five, I had zero polyps and my colon was clean as a whistle. One of the reasons why was my daily consumption of water. It is not something that you can skimp on and expect to live a long life. I have read about doctors saying that a lack of sleep shortens lives, but I would bet that bad water consumption is just as deadly.

If you are not getting 32 ounces of pure water daily, or if that water is contaminated, then you are putting stress on your system. More than that, you are impacting your immune system and limiting your life extension potential.

Believe it or not, water consumption is just as important as the nutrients that you put in your body, or the exercise and rest that you get on a daily basis. You should take your water consumption just as seriously as these other lifestyle choices.

So, for liquid consumption, water should be your primary intake. In fact, on most days, ideally, that should be your primary beverage. Moreover, if you can add fresh-squeezed lemon juice, that is even better. I nearly always include a quarter slice of lemon in my water at dinner. Lemon is a magical fruit that can help you maintain a neutral pH level.

I highly recommend that you quit caffeine. This will be discussed more in the next chapter. There is no reason to drink stimulants on a daily basis. Some green teas and herbal teas do have significant nutritional benefits, but keep the caffeine limited.

Sodas, or anything with sugar or artificial sweeteners are not conducive to life extension. Stay away.

Chapter Six: Drink Well

Fruit drinks need to be treated with caution. First, avoid any with added sugar or artificial sweeteners. Second, keep your consumption to eight ounces or less. These drinks contain high amounts of sugar, even if they are 100% fruit juice. When you drink a glass of orange juice, once you exceed eight ounces, you are eating multiple oranges. Also, unless a fruit drink is freshly squeezed, the nutritional value is reduced.

Note that dried fruit is a lot like fruit drinks, in that they are very high in sugar content. I would not consider dried fruit as a health food for this reason. I do enjoy raisins and apricots, but I tend to limit my dried fruit intake.

Juicing and blending smoothies are ideal ways to increase your nutritional intake and boost your immune system. Both are different, so I will discuss them separately.

Juicing is done with special juicing machines, and not blenders. Juicing machines have the ability to squeeze out enzymes and high nutritional content from fruits and vegetables. I have two different types of juicing machines. One type uses a fast spinning blade that is noisy, and you have to force in the food using a plunger. The other type sucks in the food and is quiet. I recommend the quiet type, which has the added benefit of being easier to clean.

Juice machines can provide miracles, and are excellent at preventative medicine. If you juice daily, you will boost your immune system significantly. This can heal chronic illnesses that other medications failed to cure. Juicing is so powerful, that it can and has cured various cancers. You can watch several documentaries about Dr. Max Gerson, and the Gerson Method that prove its efficacy. While you likely don't have cancer or a chronic illness, you can still use juicing for boosting your immune system.

Another documentary to watch is *Fat, Sick and Nearly Dead*. Joe Cross used juicing to not only heal himself without medication, but he achieved a level of health he never dreamed possible. He has transformed an untold number of lives through his documentary.

I consider juicing to be nutrition on steroids. Some people think that everyone should juice, but I'm not in that group. I do think it is very useful for good health, but the secret to longevity is being consistent with *all* aspects of life extension. Nutrition is only one aspect and will not create life extension on its own. For that reason, I think a quality blender to make smoothies is probably sufficient.

I do like to juice a few times a year to give myself a nutritional bump, and an annual digestive cleaning, but doing it on a regular basis seems like overkill when you are already healthy.

Creating fresh fruit and vegetable smoothies, including many of the superfoods that I listed in the previous chapter, is quite sufficient for boosting your nutrition. Plus, when you drink smoothies, you get all of the fiber that is removed when you use juicing machines. If I had something to do with all of my leftover fiber, I would probably juice more.

I have a friend who has a nutritional smoothie every morning for breakfast. She loads it with superfoods. I highly recommend this for breakfast. Currently, I still prefer whole grain or oat cereal for breakfast because it gives me the energy that I prefer. But smoothies for breakfast make a lot of sense.

Chapter Seven

NO DRUGS OR CHEMICALS

Humans love their drugs. Alcohol is a huge business, as is nicotine, and caffeine. All three are billion dollar industries. Marijuana is also becoming very popular, with state after state legalizing it. Caffeine might be the most abused drug of all. I wonder how many people use caffeine to feel good in the morning and alcohol to feel good at night?

Ideally, you want to exclude drugs from your body, if your goal is life extension. Although, it's okay to consume drugs in moderation and still achieve a long life. The key is not to make it a daily habit. You need to treat drugs similarly to the way you approach nutrition. It's okay to have a piece of cake once in a while, but it's not something you want to do on a daily basis.

If you eat well and exercise regularly, and then consistently consume drugs, that is counterproductive to your goal of life extension. Drugs shock the system and put stress on the natural state of well-being. The body is resilient enough to handle a daily cup of coffee or a nightly glass of wine with very little residual impact. However, over time, the stress impacted on the body adds up and reduces our lifespan.

There is a common misconception that a daily cup of coffee or a nightly glass of wine is good for you. It is true that both contain polyphenols, which are good for you. However, asking your body to adapt to your drug of choice is not good for life extension. Ideally, your body wants to maintain a state of well-being. And trust me when I say that, when you speed up (caffeine) or slow down (alcohol) your system, that is not a state of well-being..

Medications are also drugs, but they require a doctor's prescription (except for over the counter drugs). These also put stress on your system. Today, our ingestion of medications has become an epidemic. A generation ago, we did not consume mass quantities of medications. Today, it's something like one in two Americans are on some form of medication. It's so bad that, if you are over fifty, then you are probably on at least one prescription. This epidemic is clearly related to what we consume.

I'm not going to list all of the medications that people are taking today. I'm going to make this simple. Medications put the same stress on the body that legal and illegal drugs do. For this reason, ideally, you do not want to consume them on a regular basis. Try whatever you can to be medication free. Do this with your doctor's help, if that is needed. I know that some people are dependent on anti-depressants and other psychological medications. Be very careful removing those from your daily routine without your doctor's help.

The goal of life extension is to maintain a state of well-being, without putting any stress on the body or mind. That is, ideally, the best way to achieve an extended life.

Chapter Eight

PLAN TO LIVE TO 100

When I was in my twenties, I made a trip to Oregon to visit a friend. As I usually do when I travel, I found a gym to do a workout. At this gym, there were several men in their seventies who were in great shape. I was stunned. I couldn't believe it. These guys had gray hair and looked old. They were well past retirement age. They were working out with weights as if they were still in the prime of their life. I made a decision right then that I was going to never stop working out, and was going to achieve what they had achieved.

I have never lost my motivation to stay in shape and remain healthy. I plan to live until I am 100, and my goal is to remain vibrant until I am eighty-eight. What I mean by vibrant is that I can still do a workout at the gym, take a three mile run, swim a mile, or perhaps help someone move into a new house. I know that eighty-eight is pushing the threshold of what is possible, but I'm going to shoot for it. I know it's possible because many people play competitive tennis until they are ninety, and many people run long distances well into their nineties.

If you go to YouTube, you can see people in their eighties and nineties doing workouts. The body can remain vibrant much longer than many believe. I think that living an active life well into your nineties is possible. This is what has kept me motivated. I truly believe that anyone who makes the right lifestyle choices can live an extended, vibrant life well past the average lifespan.

I say that I plan to live to 100 and be vibrant until I am eighty-eight, but that only tells part of the story. My plan includes lifestyles choices which ensure that I succeed. On a daily basis, I make choices that ensure my success. For instance, rarely do I stay up past midnight. When I book an airline ticket, I try to avoid an early flight that might cause me to lose sleep. When I travel, I normally make trips to grocery stores instead of eating only at restaurants. Plus, when I'm on the road, I think about getting exercise and not skipping too many workouts. When I eat out or eat with friends and family, I make sure not to consume too much toxic food. Rarely do I travel without supplements.

I've been doing this type of daily longevity planning for over thirty years. It's a lifestyle of health, but also a lifestyle of longevity. Basically, you start living a certain way and it becomes who you are. Everything that has to do with health and longevity becomes part of your life.

I know one family whom I have visited a lot over the years. Recently, the family's mother said, "You never eat. I've never seen you eat." And this is a lady I've known for over thirty years. The reason why she never saw me eat is that I rarely snack. If I come to visit someone for a few hours, I usually do not come to eat. Instead, I usually drink water, if anything.

So, the bottom line is that you have to be serious about your daily longevity plans. You have to stick with the plan and your lifestyle choices. If you are going to exercise a little bit, eat well occasionally, take supplements once in a while, and mostly avoid drugs, that's not going to work. If that is the lifestyle you choose, then you will be relying on good genes and luck to live a long life, or to be vibrant into your eighties.

You can take luck out of the equation and extend your life proactively. Start with diet and exercise, and see if those are daily lifestyle choices you can live with. From there, you can include the rest of what I have explained in this book.

Chapter Eight: Plan to Live to 100

There are a few things that I do that I think promote well-being and vibrancy. These are good habits that I recommend. The first one is taking two showers daily. You may think this is an odd habit. I started doing it in my early twenties when I joined a gym. I would go to the gym after work, which forced me to take a second shower. After doing this routine for about a decade, I found that those second showers were stimulating and had a positive effect on my well-being. Moreover, they became habit-forming.

Today, I nearly always take a shower in the morning and then another one in the afternoon or before dinner. I've been doing this for more than thirty years. I can't explain why I think it is healthy, but I know in my gut that it is. If you Google health benefits from taking a shower, there are many. Taking that second shower is beneficial, in my opinion.

A couple of tidbits about showers. I prefer Ivory bar soap. I have used it for decades and it seems to be beneficial to my skin. Also, if you can bear it, a cold shower is very invigorating. Try one and see if you can tell the difference in your day. I had to do this once because the hot water was out, and I was surprised by how much better I felt.

The next thing I do is common sense, but I'll mention it anyway. Take care of your teeth. Brush twice a day and floss once a day. Plus, have your teeth cleaned twice a year. Do not neglect your teeth.

I have two final habits that I recommend for your well-being. The first is a colon cleanse. If you eat meat, then you will want to do these quarterly, or three times a year. I do them twice a year. I use a colon cleanse powder that I buy online. There are different brands to choose from, but they usually all taste bad. I mix it with POM blueberry-pomegranate juice and it still has a very strong peppery taste, but it is okay with the sweet fruit juice.

My final habit is, again, somewhat odd, but highly recommended. It is an ear wax cleaning. I do these every two or three years because it takes a while for the wax to build up after a good cleaning. You can purchase an ear wax removal kit from your local pharmacy. There are several brands and they are all about the same. The kit comes with three things: a dropper of a liquid solution, a rubber bubble syringe, and wax ear plugs. You place five to ten drops in each ear, then after a few minutes, you use the syringe to rinse out your ears with warm water. These kits are an excellent way to remove any wax buildup.

When you visit your doctor, have them check your ears for any wax buildup. They can tell you very quickly if your cleaning routine is working. Don't be surprised if they find some wax buildup, because nearly everyone has some. If it gets bad enough, it can impact your hearing. I thought I had lost some hearing in one of my ears and it was wax buildup!

Chapter Nine

Extreme Methods

There are a few other methods that people are currently using to obtain life extension. These are methods that I do not include in my lifestyle choices, but you may want to pursue them.

The first one is low calorie consumption. If you consistently under-eat, your body tends to age slower. It turns out that there is some scientific proof supporting this method. They tested this on both rats and mice, and they increased their lifespan by an additional thirty percent. That's a huge increase, and the reason why many people are trying it today.

If you are a highly intense, type A personality, with a goal of aging slower, this may be a good method for you to try. Often, it is done in conjunction with fasting. I have found that fasting is not easy to do. If you want a difficult challenge, then a low-calorie diet, in conjunction with fasting, is the ticket for you. Good luck.

The next method is a bit extreme and costly. It requires that you do blood transfusions using blood from someone under twenty-five. What! Yes, this is currently being done and it is legal. It is popular with the millionaire crowd in Silicon Valley.

Why would someone do a blood transfusion to extend their life? Well, again, it is based on science. They did this with animals and found that it not only had a life extension quality, but also a rejuvenation effect that reversed aging. Now, you can see the appeal. It sounds creepy, but if you could reverse aging and have a few extra bucks in the bank.... My concern is the potential side effects. Is it really a free ride to living longer?

Another method that is expensive and becoming more common is stem cell injections. There are doctors who will re-inject your own stem cells for the purpose of life extension. I don't think we've heard the end of this.

The last method is the holy grail, which is an anti-aging supplement, or perhaps even a reverse aging supplement. I think these exist, or will exist in the future. It's possible that they exist today, but are very expensive and only available to insiders, such as millionaires and billionaires.

One supplement to research is C60, also called Carbon 60. In 2012, clinical tests feeding rats C60 in olive oil extended their lifespan by up to 90%. It appears to have several benefits: slower aging, more energy, improved memory, increased strength, less fatigue, and reduced stress. It seems like the holy grail, but there could be unknown effects.

Dr. Todd Ovokaitys is working on enhancing nutrients using lasers that is very intriguing.

Google has funded an anti-aging company called Calico with $1.5 billion, hiring a team of PhD researchers. Not only do the founders of Google want to extend their lives, but they also want to develop a product to make money. I'm sure there are many other researchers working on life extension supplements, with billions being spent on research. Here is Calico's mission statement:

> Calico is a research and development company whose mission is to harness advanced technologies to increase our understanding of the biology that controls lifespan.

In our lifetime, I expect there to be many newly discovered anti-aging products released. If you are already living a life extension lifestyle, and someone comes out with an anti-aging supplement, it may add several years to your life. You will likely get a boost that others may not because your body is already in a state of

Chapter Nine: Extreme Methods

longevity. In fact, I would not be surprised if I live well beyond 100 from these developments. It's not as crazy as it sounds.

After I was finished writing this book, I heard Dave Asprey give an interview. I actually considered not publishing my book after reading his book titled, *Head Strong*. He is the true professional when it comes to life extension. His goal is to live until 180 years of age. That was not a typo. His passion around life extension is second to none.

Because his goal is so extreme, so are many of his methods. Yes, he incorporates many of the things I have written about, and then more. In many respects, his focus is two-pronged, targeted at both cellular energy and human longevity health. He lives nearly every breath to ensure his mitochondria are at optimal health. The amount of money, time, and experimentation he invests in his longevity is phenomenal.

If you are into extreme methods, then definitively read his book. As much as I pushed supplements, I am nowhere close to the amount of supplements he recommends and uses. His methods and recommendations are controversial, to say the least. For instance, he recommends a high-vegetable/high-fat diet. That's not something I can handle. Plus, he strongly recommends drinking two to five cups of coffee per day. As you know, I consider caffeine a drug, so that didn't sit well with me. And if you are convinced that saturated fat is bad for you, then you might not like his approach. However, it does work for him, and amazingly well.

I still recommend his book for some of his insights, along with many of what he calls biohacks, which are his unusual methods of achieving optimal energy levels. He equates optimum energy levels with optimum health, but I'm not so sure they correlate one to one. However, I guarantee you will learn something new. It's loaded with a lot of science and twenty-five pages of footnotes. I learned a lot, although I don't know how much of it I will apply to my life. His methods are about living well beyond 100, but my objective isn't as lofty. I'll be quite satisfied to live vibrantly until I am ninety.

BOOK REVIEW REQUEST

If you enjoyed this book and think that others would benefit from reading it, please write a review. Most readers rely on reviews to make their decision. It's sort of a catch-22 for me as a writer. I need reviews to sell books, but I need to sell books to get reviews. If you could help, that would be much appreciated.

www.ingramcontent.com/pod-product-compliance
Lightning Source LLC
Chambersburg PA
CBHW071122030426
42336CB00013BA/2165